SIMPLE STRAIGHT FORWARD COOKING RECIPES FOR ALL ENDOMORPHS

enjoy your meal

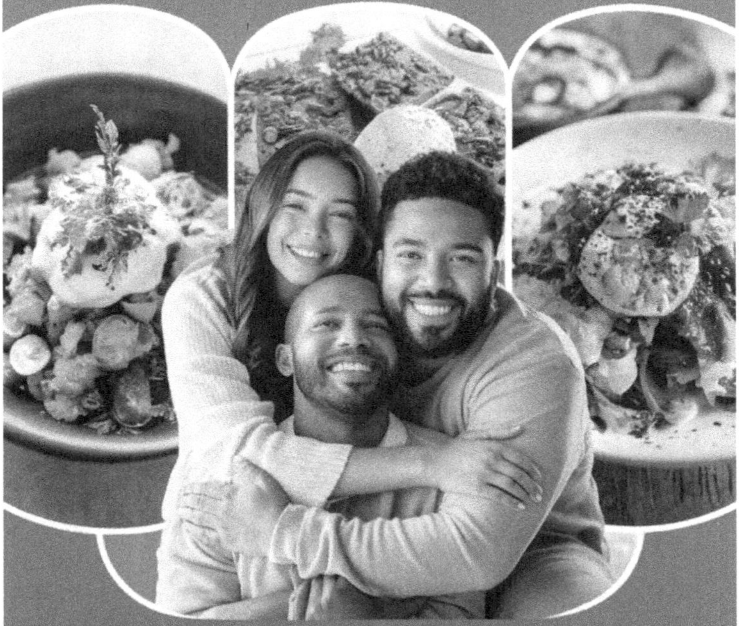

Endomorph Diet

Boost Metabolism, Shed Fat, and Achieve Lasting Wellness with a 28-Day Meal Plan, Delicious Recipes, and Proven Strategies for Your Body Type

Written by Mary Williams

Gratitude speech

Thank you. From the bottom of my heart, thank you for picking up this book. Your trust in me to help you on your health journey means the world. This book is my gift to you, but the true gift is yours to give yourself – a healthier, happier you. Let's transform together, one page at a time. Thank you.

About the Book

Your Guide to Health and Well-being as an Endomorph

This book is designed to empower you, an endomorph, to take control of your health and create a sustainable lifestyle that works for your unique body type.

Here's what you'll find inside:

 * **Understanding Endomorphs:** Explore the characteristics of endomorphs, including body shape, hormonal profile, and metabolic tendencies.
 * **Dietary Strategies for Success:** Discover how to manage your weight through balanced meals, portion control, and macronutrient intake tailored for endomorphs.

* Delicious Recipe Ideas: Find healthy and satisfying breakfast, lunch, dinner, and snack options to keep you fueled throughout the day.

* Exercise for Endomorphs: Learn how to incorporate strength training, HIIT workouts, and moderate-intensity cardio to boost your metabolism and overall fitness.

* Mindful Eating Practices: Cultivate a healthy relationship with food through mindful eating techniques to combat cravings and emotional eating.

* Tracking Progress and Making Adjustments: Discover strategies for monitoring your progress and adapting your plan for long-term success.

More than just a weight-loss guide, this book is a comprehensive resource for endomorphs seeking to:

* Manage weight and improve body composition

* Increase energy levels and feel your best

* Develop healthy and sustainable habits

* Embrace a love for movement and physical activity

With this book as your companion, you'll embark on a journey of self-discovery and empowerment. Take charge of your health and create a life that is both fulfilling and sustainable.

Contents

Breakfast Recipes.. 43

Lunch Recipes.. 46

Dinner Recipes... 48

Added Recipes..49

quick and easy meal that's perfect for busy weeknights... 50

Snack Ideas...51

practical tips to nudge their metabolism in a healthy way:..52

How to incorporate exercise into an endomorph fitness plan..54

Cultivating Mindful Eating Habits............................ 56

Introduction

Welcome! **This book is designed to be your guide to health and well-being as an endomorph.** It will equip you with the knowledge and tools to create a sustainable lifestyle that supports your unique body type. We'll explore the characteristics of endomorphs, dive into the importance of diet and exercise, and provide a personalized 28-day meal plan with delicious recipes to jumpstart your journey. By the end, you'll have the strategies and motivation you need to achieve lasting results and feel your best.

Understanding Endomorph Body Type

The endomorph body type is characterized by a slower metabolism, a rounder body shape, and a higher percentage of body fat. These characteristics are partly influenced by genetics, which means endomorphs may be naturally predisposed to store fat more easily. However, this doesn't define your potential for health and fitness.

Endomorphs also have some advantages. They tend to have a strong and sturdy body type and may find it easier to build muscle mass. The key to success for endomorphs lies in understanding how their bodies work and creating a personalized approach to diet and exercise that promotes long-term health and well-being.

The Importance of Diet for Endomorphs

Diet plays a crucial role in achieving and maintaining a healthy weight for endomorphs.

Due to their slower metabolism, endomorphs need to be mindful of calorie intake and focus on consuming foods that promote satiety, regulate blood sugar, and support metabolism.

Here's why diet is essential:
 * Manages Blood Sugar: Endomorphs may be more prone to blood sugar spikes and crashes.

A balanced diet rich in complex carbohydrates, protein, and healthy fats helps regulate blood sugar, preventing energy dips and cravings.

 * Boosts Metabolism: Certain foods can act as natural metabolism boosters. Protein requires more energy for digestion compared to carbohydrates or fats. Including lean protein sources throughout the day can help increase calorie burning.

 * Promotes Satiety: Feeling full and satisfied after meals is key to avoiding unhealthy snacking. Fiber-rich

foods like vegetables, fruits, and whole grains promote satiety and keep you feeling fuller for longer.

* Provides Essential Nutrients: A well-rounded diet ensures your body gets the vitamins, minerals, and antioxidants it needs to function optimally.

In the next section, "Creating a 28-Day Meal Plan," we'll explore how to design a meal plan that incorporates these dietary principles to support your weight management goals and overall health.

Creating a 28-Day Meal Plan

A 28-day meal plan can be a valuable tool for endomorphs to jumpstart their health journey and establish sustainable eating habits. Here's what we'll cover in this section:

* Meal Plan Principles: We'll delve into the core principles of creating a meal plan for endomorphs, including portion control, macronutrient balance (fats, carbohydrates, protein), and meal frequency.

* Sample Meal Plan: We'll provide a sample 28-day meal plan as a blueprint. This will include breakfast, lunch, dinner, and snack options, showcasing variety and portion sizes.

* Customizing Your Plan: We'll discuss how to personalize the sample meal plan to your preferences, dietary needs, and calorie requirements.

* Meal Prep Tips: We'll offer valuable tips for meal prepping to save time and ensure you have healthy meals readily available throughout the week.

By following these guidelines and utilizing the sample meal plan, you can create a personalized approach to healthy eating that supports your weight management goals and keeps you energized throughout the day.

Recipe 1. Chicken and Vegetable Stir Fry

Ingredients:
- 1 chicken breast, sliced
- 1 cup broccoli florets
- 1 cup sliced carrots
- 1 cup sliced bell peppers
- 2 cloves garlic, minced
- 1 inch ginger, grated
- 2 tbsp low-sodium soy sauce
- 1 tsp sesame oil

Method:
1. Slice the chicken breast into thin strips. Chop vegetables.
2. Heat a large skillet over medium-high heat with 1 tsp sesame oil.
3. Add chicken and stir fry for 5 minutes until no longer pink. Remove from the skillet.
4. Add remaining 1 tsp sesame oil to skillet. Add vegetables and stir fry for 5 more minutes.
5. Return chicken to skillet. Add soy sauce and garlic. Toss to coat. Cook for 2 more minutes.

Cooking Time: 12 minutes
Nutrition (per serving): 250 calories, 7g fat, 32g protein, 15g carbs

Recipe 2. Black Bean Salad

Ingredients:
- 1 (15oz) can black beans, rinsed and drained
- 1 cup corn kernels, fresh or frozen
- 1 tomato, diced
- 1/2 red onion, diced
- 1/4 cup fresh cilantro, chopped
- 2 tbsp olive oil
- 2 tbsp lime juice
- 1/2 tsp ground cumin
- Salt and pepper to taste

Method:
1. In a large bowl, combine black beans, corn, tomato and red onion.
2. In a small bowl, whisk together olive oil, lime juice, cumin and salt and pepper.
3. Pour dressing over bean mixture and toss to coat. Top with cilantro.

Cooking Time: 5 minutes

Nutrition (per serving): 250 calories, 8g fat, 10g protein, 38g carbs

Recipe 3. Chicken Parmesan

Ingredients:
- 4 chicken cutlets
- 1/2 cup almond flour
- 1 egg
- 1/2 cup marinara sauce
- 1 cup shredded part-skim mozzarella

Method:
1. Preheat the oven to 400°F and grease a baking dish.
2. Place almond flour in a shallow dish. In another dish, whisk egg.
3. Dredge chicken in flour, then egg, then back in flour to coat.
4. Place breaded chicken in a baking dish. Top with marinara sauce and cheese.
5. Bake 20-25 minutes until chicken is cooked through and cheese is melted.

Cooking Time: 25 minutes
Nutrition (per serving): 350 calories, 15g fat, 42g protein, 8g carbs

Recipe 4. Turkey Chili

Ingredients:
- 1 lb ground turkey
- 1 can red kidney beans, rinsed and drained
- 1 can diced tomatoes
- 1 cup vegetable or chicken broth
- 1 onion, diced
- 2 cloves garlic, minced
- 1 tsp chili powder
- 1/2 tsp cumin
- Salt and pepper to taste

Method:
1. In a large pot, cook ground turkey over medium-high heat until no longer pink.
2. Add onions and garlic and cook for 5 more minutes.
3. Stir in beans, tomatoes, broth and spices. Bring to a boil then reduce heat and simmer for 15 mins.

Cooking Time: 20 minutes

Nutrition (per serving): 250 calories, 6g fat, 28g protein, 20g carbs

Recipe 5. Salmon with Green Beans

Ingredients:
- 4 salmon filets
- 1 lb green beans, trimmed
- 2 tbsp olive oil
- Salt and pepper
- Lemon wedges

Method:
1. Preheat the oven to 400°F and line a baking sheet with foil.
2. Place salmon on foil and brush with 1 tbsp olive oil. Season with salt and pepper.
3. Toss green beans with remaining 1 tbsp olive oil on another part of the baking sheet.
4. Roast for 15-20 minutes until the salmon is opaque and the beans are tender. Serve with lemon.

Cooking Time: 20 minutes

Nutrition (per serving): 300 calories, 15g fat, 32g protein, 8g carbs

Recipe 6. Tuna Noodle Salad

Ingredients:
- 8 oz whole wheat pasta
- 2 (5oz) cans tuna in water, drained
- 1 cup cherry tomatoes, halved
- 1/2 cucumber, chopped
- 1/4 cup red onion, diced
- 1/4 cup light mayonnaise
- 2 tbsp lemon juice
- Salt and pepper to taste

Method:
1. Cook pasta according to package instructions. Drain and rinse under cold water.
2. In a large bowl, combine pasta, tuna, tomatoes, cucumber and onion.
3. In a small bowl, whisk mayonnaise, lemon juice, and salt and pepper.
4. Pour dressing over pasta mixture and toss to coat.

Cooking Time: 15 minutes

Nutrition (per serving): 350 calories, 8g fat, 28g protein, 45g carbs

Recipe 7. Beef and Broccoli Stir Fry

Ingredients:
- 12 oz beef sirloin, sliced thin
- 1 bag broccoli florets
- 1 cup bell peppers, sliced
- 2 cloves garlic, minced
- 2 tbsp oyster sauce
- 1 tbsp soy sauce
- 1/2 tbsp sesame oil

Method:
1. In a skillet over high heat, stir fry beef for 2-3 minutes until browned. Remove from the skillet.
2. Add sesame oil to the skillet. Add broccoli and peppers and stir fry for 4 minutes.
3. Push vegetables to the sides of the skillet. Pour oyster sauce in the center and let it sizzle.
4. Add beef and soy sauce back to the skillet. Toss to coat and cook 2 more minutes.

Cooking Time: 12 minutes

Nutrition (per serving): 350 calories, 12g fat, 42g protein, 15g carbs

Recipe 8. Poached Salmon Salad

Ingredients:
- 4 salmon filets
- 2 cups green beans, trimmed
- 2 cups spinach
- 1 avocado, diced
- 1 lemon, juiced
- 2 tbsp olive oil
- Salt and pepper

Method:
1. Bring a skillet of water to a simmer. Poach salmon for 8-10 minutes until opaque.
2. Steam green beans for 5 minutes until crisp-tender.
3. Toss green beans and spinach with avocado, lemon juice and olive oil.
4. Top salad with poached salmon and season with salt and pepper.

Cooking Time: 15 minutes

Nutrition (per serving): 450 calories, 28g fat, 32g protein, 13g carbs

Recipe 9. Chicken Pasta Primavera

Ingredients:
- 8 oz whole wheat pasta
- 1 lb chicken breasts, cubed
- 1 bag frozen primavera veggies
- 1 jar alfredo sauce
- Salt and pepper

Method:
1. Cook pasta according to package instructions.
2. In a skillet over medium heat, sauté chicken until no longer pink. Remove from the skillet.
3. In the same skillet, heat veggies until tender.
4. Return chicken to skillet. Add alfredo sauce and toss to coat thoroughly.
5. Serve vegetable-chicken mixture over cooked pasta.

Cooking Time: 25 minutes

Nutrition (per serving): 450 calories, 14g fat, 42g protein, 45g carbs

:

Recipe 10. Turkey Meatloaf

Ingredients:
- 1 lb ground turkey
- 1/2 cup grated carrots
- 1/3 cup oats
- 1 egg
- 1/4 cup ketchup
- 1 onion, diced
- Salt and pepper to taste

Method:
1. Preheat the oven to 375°F.
2. Mix all ingredients together in a bowl until well combined.
3. Form into a loaf and place in a baking dish.
4. Bake for 50-60 minutes until cooked through.

Cooking Time: 1 hour

Nutrition (per serving): 150 calories, 4g fat, 18g protein, 10g carbs

Recipe 11. Shrimp and Vegetable Stir Fry

Ingredients:
- 1 lb shrimp, peeled and deveined
- 2 cups assorted veggies (broccoli, carrots, peppers)
- 2 cloves garlic, minced
- 1 inch ginger, grated
- 2 tbsp oyster sauce
- 1 tbsp rice vinegar
- 1 tsp sesame oil

Method:
1. Stir fry shrimp until pink. Remove from the skillet.
2. Add sesame oil to the skillet. Cook veggies for 5 mins.
3. Push veggies to the side of the skillet. Add oyster sauce and vinegar to the center.
4. Add shrimp back to the skillet and toss to coat. Cook for 2 more mins.

Cooking Time: 15 minutes

Nutrition (per serving): 200 calories, 3.5g fat, 29g protein, 12g carbs

Recipe 12. Sheet Pan Chicken and Veggies

Ingredients:
- 4 chicken breasts
- 2 potatoes, diced
- 2 cups Brussels sprouts, halved
- 1 onion, sliced
- 2 tbsp olive oil
- Salt and pepper

Method:
1. Preheat the oven to 400°F and line a baking sheet with foil.
2. Toss potatoes, Brussels sprouts and onion with olive oil on a baking sheet.
3. Season chicken with salt and pepper and place on a sheet.
4. Roast 25-30 minutes, flipping halfway, until chicken is cooked through.

Cooking Time: 30 minutes

Nutrition (per serving): 350 calories, 10g fat, 42g protein, 20g carbs

Recipe 13. Tuna Casserole

Ingredients:
- 8 oz whole wheat elbow pasta
- 2 (5oz) cans tuna, drained
- 1 cup frozen peas
- 1 can condensed cream of celery soup
- 1/2 cup 2% milk
- 1/4 cup shredded cheddar cheese

Method:
1. Preheat the oven to 350°F and grease a 9x13 casserole dish.
2. Cook pasta until al dente. Drain and return to the pot.
3. Add tuna, peas, soup and milk. Mix well.
4. Transfer pasta mixture to prepared dish. Top with cheese.
5. Bake for 30 minutes until hot and bubbly.

Cooking Time: 35 minutes

Nutrition (per serving): 300 calories, 7g fat, 28g protein, 32g carbs

Recipe 14. Pork Stir Fry

Ingredients:
- 12 oz pork tenderloin, sliced
- 1 bag coleslaw mix
- 1 bell pepper, sliced
- 2 cloves garlic, minced
- 2 tbsp low-sodium soy sauce
- 1 tbsp rice vinegar
- 1 tsp sesame oil

Method:
1. Stir fry pork over high heat until no longer pink. Remove from the skillet.
2. Add sesame oil to the skillet. Cook vegetables for 5 mins.
3. Return pork to skillet. Add soy sauce, vinegar. Toss to coat.
4. Cook for 2 more mins until the vegetables are tender.

Cooking Time: 15 minutes

Nutrition (per serving): 250 calories, 8g fat, 29g protein, 10g carbs

Recipe 15. Veggie and Hummus Pitas

Ingredients:
- 2 whole wheat pita breads
- 1 cup mixed veggies (carrots, bell peppers, cucumber)
- 1/2 cup hummus
- Lettuce, sliced tomato

Method:
1. Slice open and split pita breads.
2. Fill each with veggies, hummus, lettuce and tomato.

No cooking required!

Nutrition (per sandwich): 300 calories, 8g fat, 10g protein, 48g carbs

Recipe 16. Chicken and Wild Rice Soup

Ingredients:
- 1 lb chicken breasts, diced
- 4 cups chicken broth
- 1 cup wild rice
- 1 cup carrots, diced
- 1 cup celery, diced
- 1 onion, diced
- 1 bay leaf
- Salt and pepper to taste

Method:
1. Add all ingredients except chicken to a soup pot and bring to a boil.
2. Reduce heat, cover and simmer 30-40 minutes until rice is tender.
3. Add chicken during the last 10 minutes of simmering.
4. Remove bay leaf before serving.

Cooking Time: 40 minutes

Nutrition (per serving): 250 calories, 3g fat, 30g protein, 26g carbs

Recipe 17. Tofu Stir Fry

Ingredients:
- 14 oz extra firm tofu, cubed
- 1 bag frozen stir fry veggies
- 2 cloves garlic, minced
- 1 inch ginger, grated
- 2 tbsp low-sodium soy sauce
- 1 tbsp rice vinegar
- 1 tsp sesame oil

Method:
1. In a skillet, stir fry tofu over med-high heat for 6-8 mins until lightly browned.
2. Add sesame oil and cook veggies for 5 mins.
3. Push veggies to sides of skillet. Add soy sauce and vinegar to the center.
4. Return tofu to the skillet and toss to coat. Cook for 2 more mins.

Cooking Time: 15 minutes

Nutrition (per serving): 250 calories, 12g fat, 18g protein, 18g carbs

Recipe 18. Cod with Potatoes and Green Beans

Ingredients:
- 4 cod filets
- 1 lb new potatoes, quartered
- 8 oz green beans, trimmed
- 2 tbsp olive oil
- Salt and pepper

Method:
1. Preheat the oven to 400°F and line a baking sheet with foil.
2. Toss potatoes and green beans with 1 tbsp olive oil on a baking sheet.
3. Season cod filets with salt and pepper and place on a baking sheet.
4. Drizzle remaining 1 tbsp olive oil over fish.
5. Roast 20-25 minutes until fish is opaque and vegetables are tender.

Cooking Time: 25 minutes

Nutrition (per serving): 300 calories, 10g fat, 32g protein, 20g carbs

Recipe 19. Quinoa Stir Fry Bowl

Ingredients:
- 1 cup quinoa
- 2 cups vegetable or chicken broth
- 1 bag frozen stir fry vegetables
- 1 lb chicken breast, cooked and diced
- 2 cloves garlic, minced
- 1 inch ginger, grated
- 2 tbsp low-sodium soy sauce

Method:
1. Bring quinoa and broth to a boil. Cover and reduce heat to low. Simmer for 15 mins.
2. Steam or stir fry vegetables until tender.
3. In a large bowl, combine quinoa, veggies and chicken.
4. Stir in garlic, ginger and soy sauce.

Cooking Time: 25 minutes

Nutrition (per serving): 400 calories, 6g fat, 37g protein, 50g carbs

Recipe 20. Tuna Casserole

Ingredients:
- 8 oz whole wheat pasta
- 2 (5oz) cans tuna, drained
- 1 cup frozen peas
- 1 cup mushroom soup
- 1/2 cup milk
- Salt and pepper to taste

Method:
1. Preheat the oven to 350°F and grease a 9x13 casserole dish.
2. Cook pasta until al dente. Drain and return to the pot.
3. Add tuna, peas, soup and milk. Mix well.
4. Transfer pasta mixture to prepared dish.
5. Bake for 30 minutes until hot and bubbly.

Cooking Time: 40 minutes

Nutrition (per serving): 350 calories, 5g fat, 28g protein, 50g carbs

Recipe 21. Sheet Pan Salmon and Vegetables

Ingredients:
- 4 salmon filets
- 2 cups Brussels sprouts, halved
- 1 lb fingerling potatoes, halved
- 1 onion, sliced
- 2 tbsp olive oil
- Salt and pepper

Method:
1. Preheat the oven to 400°F and line a baking sheet with foil.
2. Toss vegetables with olive oil on a baking sheet.
3. Season salmon filets and place on top of vegetables.
4. Roast for 20-25 minutes until the salmon is opaque and the vegetables are tender.

Cooking Time: 25 minutes

Nutrition (per serving): 400 calories, 18g fat, 32g protein, 25g carbs

Recipe 22. *Lentil Soup*

Ingredients:
- 1 cup dried lentils
- 6 cups vegetable or chicken broth
- 1 onion, diced
- 3 carrots, sliced
- 2 cloves garlic, minced
- 1 tsp thyme
- Salt and pepper

Method:
1. Add all ingredients to a pot and bring to a boil.
2. Reduce heat and simmer for 30 minutes, until lentils are tender.
3. Use an immersion blender to slightly mash some of the lentils.

Cooking Time: 30 minutes

Nutrition (per serving): 250 calories, 1.5g fat, 18g protein, 40g carbs

Recipe 23. Chicken and Vegetable Fried Rice

Ingredients:
- 1 lb chicken breast, diced
- 3 cups cooked brown rice
- 1 bag frozen Asian vegetables
- 2 eggs, beaten
- 2 tbsp low-sodium soy sauce
- Sesame oil

Method:
1. Stir fry chicken until it is no longer pink. Remove from work.
2. Add sesame oil and stir fry eggs to make scrambled eggs.
3. Add vegetables and rice and stir fry for 5 minutes.
4. Return chicken to wok. Stir in soy sauce. Cook for 2 more minutes.

Cooking Time: 20 minutes

Nutrition (per serving): 400 calories, 7g fat, 42g protein, 43g carbs

Recipe 24. Zucchini Noodle Stir Fry

Ingredients:
- 4 zucchini, spiralized
- 1 lb chicken or shrimp, sliced
- 1 red bell pepper, sliced
- 1 bag coleslaw mix
- 2 cloves garlic, minced
- 1 tbsp low-sodium soy sauce
- Sesame oil

Method:
1. Stir fry meat until it is no longer pink. Remove from work.
2. Add sesame oil and stir fry vegetables for 5 minutes.
3. Return meat to work. Stir in soy sauce. Cook for 2 more minutes.

Cooking Time: 15 minutes

Nutrition (per serving): 300 calories, 6g fat, 42g protein, 15g carbs

Recipe 25. Chili Lime Chicken

Ingredients:
- 4 chicken breasts
- 1 lime, juiced
- 1 tbsp chili powder
- 1 tsp cumin
- 1/2 tsp oregano
- Salt and pepper
- Sautéed vegetables

Method:
1. Sprinkle chicken with lime juice, chili powder, cumin, oregano and salt/pepper.
2. Heat skillet over medium and cook chicken for 5-7 minutes per side until cooked through.
3. Serve chicken with sautéed vegetables.

Cooking Time: 15 minutes

Nutrition: 250 calories, 3 g fat, 46 g protein, 3 g carbs

Recipe 26. Shrimp and Grits

Ingredients:
- 14 oz shrimp, peeled and deveined
- 1 cup stone ground grits
- 2 slices bacon
- 1 cup shredded cheese
- Garlic, salt, pepper

Method:
1. Cook grits according to the package.
2. Cook bacon and shrimp with garlic until shrimp are pink.
3. Pour shrimp/bacon mixture over grits and top with cheese.

Cooking Time: 30 minutes

Nutrition: 400 calories, 15 g fat, 35 g protein, 30 g carbs

Recipe 27. Thai Turkey Lettuce Wraps

Ingredients:
- 1 lb ground turkey
- 1 cup coleslaw mix
- 1/4 cup peanut sauce
- 8 butter lettuce leaves

Method:
1. Cook turkey until browned and vegetables are tender.
2. Place turkey mixture in lettuce leaves and top with peanut sauce.

Cooking Time: 15 minutes

Nutrition: 300 calories, 12 g fat, 28 g protein, 12 g carbs

Recipe 28. Vegetable Frittata

Ingredients:
- 6 eggs
- 1 cup chopped vegetables (peppers, spinach, onions etc.)
- 1/4 cup shredded cheese
- 1 tbsp olive oil
- Salt and pepper

Method:

1. Preheat the oven to 350°F.

2. Heat oil in an oven-safe skillet over medium. Sauté vegetables until softened.

3. In a bowl, whisk eggs with salt and pepper. Pour into the skillet with vegetables.

4. Cook 3-5 minutes until bottom sets. Sprinkle it with cheese.

5. Bake for 15-20 minutes until set. Allow to cool slightly before slicing.

Nutrition (per 1/4 frittata):
150 calories, 10g fat, 10g protein, 3g carbs

This frittata recipe is very versatile - you can change up the veggies and cheese each time. It's a perfect make-ahead breakfast or meal prep option. The eggs and veggies provide good protein and nutrients to keep you full as an endomorph-friendly breakfast or snack.

Breakfast Recipes

Here are some breakfast recipe ideas for endomorphs that focus on protein, healthy fats, and fiber to keep you feeling satisfied throughout the morning:

Power Greens Scramble

This protein-packed scramble is loaded with vitamins, minerals, and healthy fats to keep you energized.

Ingredients:
 * 2 large eggs
 * 1 cup chopped spinach
 * ½ cup chopped mushrooms
 * ¼ cup crumbled feta cheese
 * 1 tablespoon olive oil
 * Salt and pepper to taste

Instructions:
 * Heat olive oil in a pan over medium heat. Add mushrooms and cook until softened, about 3 minutes.
 * Push the mushrooms to one side of the pan and add the eggs. Scramble the eggs until cooked through.
 * Stir in the spinach and feta cheese until heated through.
 * Season with salt and pepper to taste.

Cooking Time: 10 minutes

Nutritional Information:

* Calories: 280
* Protein: 18g
* Carbs: 8g
* Fat: 16g

Variations:

 * For a vegetarian option, omit the feta cheese and add ¼ cup crumbled tofu.

 * Add other chopped vegetables like bell peppers, onions, or tomatoes for extra flavor and nutrients.

 * For a heartier scramble, serve with a whole-wheat toast or a slice of whole-grain bread.

Greek Yogurt Parfait with Berries and Nuts

This parfait is a great source of protein and healthy fats, and the berries add a touch of sweetness and fiber.
Ingredients:
 * 1 cup plain Greek yogurt
 * ½ cup mixed berries
 * ¼ cup chopped nuts (almonds, walnuts, or pecans)
 * 1 tablespoon chia seeds (optional)
 * Drizzle of honey (optional)
Instructions:
 * Layer the Greek yogurt, berries, nuts, and chia seeds in a parfait glass.
 * Drizzle with honey for a touch of sweetness (optional).
Cooking Time: 5 minutes
Nutritional Information:
 * Calories: 300
 * Protein: 20g
 * Carbs: 25g
 * Fat: 10g

Lunch Recipes

*L*et's move on to Lunch Recipes. Here are some ideas that prioritize lean protein, complex carbohydrates, and healthy fats to keep you energized for the afternoon:

Tuna Salad with Whole-Wheat Wrap

This recipe is a quick and easy lunch option that's packed with protein and healthy fats.

Ingredients:
 * 1 can (5 oz) tuna in water, drained
 * ½ cup chopped celery
 * ¼ cup chopped red onion
 * 2 tablespoons light mayonnaise
 * 1 tablespoon lemon juice
 * Salt and pepper to taste
 * 1 whole-wheat wrap

Instructions:
 * In a bowl, combine tuna, celery, red onion, mayonnaise, lemon juice, salt, and pepper.
 * Spread the mixture onto a whole-wheat wrap and roll up tightly.

Cooking Time: 10 minutes

Nutritional Information:
 * Calories: 350
 * Protein: 30g
 * Carbs: 30g
 * Fat: 10g

Lentil Soup with Whole-Grain Bread

This hearty soup is a great source of protein and fiber, and it's also very affordable.

Ingredients:
 * 1 cup brown lentils, rinsed
 * 4 cups vegetable broth
 * 1 cup chopped carrots
 * 1 cup chopped celery
 * 1/2 cup chopped onion
 * 1 clove garlic, minced
 * 1 teaspoon dried thyme
 * 1/2 teaspoon ground cumin
 * Salt and pepper to taste
 * 2 slices whole-grain bread

Instructions:
 * In a large pot, combine lentils, vegetable broth, carrots, celery, onion, garlic, thyme, cumin, salt, and pepper.
 * Bring to a boil, then reduce heat and simmer for 30 minutes, or until lentils are tender.
 * Serve with whole-grain bread.

Cooking Time: 40 minutes

Nutritional Information:
 * Calories: 400
 * Protein: 18g
 * Carbs: 60g
 * Fat: 10g

Dinner Recipes

*L*et's delve into dinner recipes that are both satisfying and promote your weight management goals. Here are some key concepts to keep in mind for endomorph-friendly dinners:

 * **Lean Protein Source**: Include a lean protein source like grilled chicken, fish, or tofu in most dinners. Protein keeps you feeling full and helps regulate blood sugar.

 * **Non-Starchy Vegetables**: Load up on non-starchy vegetables like broccoli, spinach, or asparagus. These are low in calories and carbohydrates but high in fiber and essential nutrients.

 * **Healthy Fats**: Don't shy away from healthy fats like olive oil, avocado, or nuts. Healthy fats promote satiety and aid in nutrient absorption.

 * **Portion Control**: Be mindful of portion sizes. Even healthy foods can contribute to weight gain if consumed in excess.

Added Recipes

Salmon with Roasted Vegetables

This dish is packed with flavor and nutrients.
Ingredients:
 * 1 salmon filet (4 oz)
 * 1 tablespoon olive oil
 * Salt and pepper to taste
 * 1 cup chopped broccoli florets
 * 1 cup chopped Brussels sprouts
 * 1/2 cup chopped red onion
 * 1 tablespoon balsamic vinegar
Instructions:
 * Preheat the oven to 400°F (200°C).
 * Toss broccoli, Brussels sprouts, and red onion with olive oil, salt, and pepper. Spread on a baking sheet.
 * Season salmon filet with salt and pepper. Place on top of the vegetables.
 * Roast for 20-25 minutes, or until salmon is cooked through and vegetables are tender-crisp.
 * Drizzle with balsamic vinegar before serving.
Chicken Stir-Fry with Brown Rice

quick and easy meal that's perfect for busy weeknights.

Ingredients:
 * 1 pound boneless, skinless chicken breasts, sliced thin
 * 2 tablespoons soy sauce
 * 1 tablespoon cornstarch
 * 1 tablespoon vegetable oil
 * 2 cups chopped mixed vegetables (broccoli, carrots, peppers)
 * 1 cup cooked brown rice

Instructions:
 * In a bowl, combine chicken, soy sauce, and cornstarch. Mix well.
 * Heat oil in a large skillet or wok over medium-high heat. Add chicken and cook until browned, about 5 minutes.
 * Add vegetables and stir-fry for 5-7 minutes, or until tender-crisp.
 * Serve over cooked brown rice.

Snack Ideas.

Here are some key principles to keep in mind for endomorph-friendly snacks:

 * Protein and Fiber: Prioritize snacks that contain protein and fiber to promote satiety and manage blood sugar levels.

 * Portion Control: Practice mindful portion control to avoid exceeding your daily calorie needs.

 * Healthy Fats: Include healthy fats like nuts, seeds, or avocado for sustained energy and nutrient absorption.

 * Natural Sugars: Opt for whole fruits over processed snacks with added sugar.

Here are some snack ideas that incorporate these principles:

 * Hard-boiled eggs with a handful of almonds
 * Sliced apple or pear with nut butter
 * Greek yogurt with berries and a sprinkle of chia seeds
 * Carrot sticks with hummus
 * Edamame pods
 * Trail mix made with nuts, seeds, and dried fruit (be mindful of portion sizes)

Remember, these are just suggestions. Feel free to get creative and explore healthy snack options that suit your preferences. In the next section, we'll discuss strategies to boost metabolism for weight management.

practical tips to nudge their metabolism in a healthy way:

1. **Strength Training:** Building muscle mass can increase your basal metabolic rate (BMR), the number of calories your body burns at rest. Strength training 2-3 times a week, targeting major muscle groups, can be highly beneficial.

2. **High-Intensity Interval Training (HIIT):** Short bursts of intense exercise followed by periods of rest can rev up your metabolism and burn more calories in less time. HIIT workouts are a time-efficient way to boost metabolism.

3. **Eat Regularly:** Skipping meals can actually slow down your metabolism. Aim for 3 balanced meals and healthy snacks throughout the day to keep your metabolism functioning optimally.

4. **Stay Hydrated:** Drinking plenty of water can improve digestion and may also play a role in metabolism. Aim for at least eight glasses of water per day.

5. **Quality Sleep:** When you're sleep deprived, your body produces more ghrelin, a hunger hormone, and less leptin, a satiety hormone. This can lead to increased calorie intake and weight gain. Prioritize 7-8 hours of quality sleep each night.

6. **Manage Stress**: Chronic stress can elevate cortisol levels, a hormone that can promote fat storage. Find healthy ways to manage stress, such as yoga, meditation, or spending time in nature.

By incorporating these strategies into your routine, you can create a sustainable approach to weight management and support a healthy metabolism.

In the next section, we'll explore how to integrate exercise effectively into your endomorph fitness plan.

How to incorporate exercise into an endomorph fitness plan.

Here are some key points to consider:
Focus on Strength Training:
 * Build Muscle Mass: As mentioned earlier, muscle burns more calories at rest than fat. Strength training 2-3 times a week, targeting major muscle groups like legs, back, chest, and shoulders, can significantly increase your basal metabolic rate (BMR).
HIIT Workouts for a Boost:
 * Short Bursts, Big Results: High-Intensity Interval Training (HIIT) involves alternating between short bursts of intense exercise and periods of rest or low-intensity activity. This style of exercise can torch calories efficiently and elevate your metabolism even after the workout.
Cardio Doesn't Get Left Behind:
 * Moderate-Intensity Cardio: While HIIT offers benefits, don't neglect moderate-intensity cardio like brisk walking, swimming, or cycling. Aim for at least 150 minutes of moderate-cardio or 75 minutes of vigorous-intensity cardio each week for overall fitness and heart health.

Find Activities You Enjoy:
 * Consistency is Key: Consistency is crucial for reaping the rewards of exercise. Choose activities you find enjoyable, whether it's hitting the gym, dancing at home, or joining a fitness class. Fun workouts are more likely to become sustainable habits.

Listen to Your Body:
 * Rest and Recovery: Don't push yourself to the point of exhaustion. Schedule rest days for recovery, and pay attention to your body's signals. If you experience pain, adjust your workout intensity or seek professional guidance.

Start Gradually and Progress:
 * Avoid Overexertion: If you're new to exercise, begin with low-impact activities and gradually increase intensity and duration as your fitness improves. This will help prevent injuries and keep you motivated.

By following these tips, you can create a well-rounded exercise routine that complements your diet and supports your weight management goals as an endomorph. In the next section, we'll delve into mindful eating techniques to enhance your weight management journey.

Cultivating Mindful Eating Habits

Mindful eating involves bringing awareness and focus to the act of eating. It's about more than just the food itself; it's about your thoughts, feelings, and physical cues surrounding food choices and consumption. Here are some key aspects of mindful eating that can benefit endomorphs:

 * **Disconnecting from Distractions**: Eat without distractions like television, phones, or work. Focus on the experience of eating and savor your food.

 * **Slow Down and Enjoy**: Eat slowly and chew your food thoroughly. This allows your body to register satiety signals, preventing overeating.

 * **Listen to Your Body Hunger Cues**: Learn to distinguish between true hunger and emotional or boredom eating. Pay attention to your body's hunger cues and eat until comfortably satisfied, not stuffed.

 * **Plan Your Meals and Snacks**: Planning meals and snacks in advance can help you make healthier choices and avoid unhealthy impulse decisions.

 * **Mindful Grocery Shopping**: Be mindful when grocery shopping. Opt for whole, unprocessed foods and limit sugary drinks and processed snacks.

* **Gratitude for Your Food**: Take a moment to appreciate the food on your plate. Consider its origin, preparation, and nourishment it provides.

By incorporating these mindful eating practices, endomorphs can gain greater control over their eating habits and make food choices that align with their weight management goals and overall well-being. In the following section, we'll tackle strategies for managing cravings and emotional eating, common hurdles for many trying to lose weight.

Understanding Cravings and Emotional Eating

Cravings and emotional eating are common obstacles for people trying to manage their weight. Endomorphs, due to their hormonal profile, may be more susceptible to cravings for high-sugar, high-fat foods. Here, we'll explore how to identify and deal with these challenges:

 * Cravings vs. Hunger: Distinguish between true hunger pangs and cravings triggered by emotions, stress, or boredom. Hunger cues are gradual, while cravings hit suddenly and often for specific foods.

 * Identify Your Triggers: Recognize the emotional triggers that lead to emotional eating. Are you reaching for comfort food when stressed, anxious, or bored? Journaling can help identify patterns.

 * Healthy Coping Mechanisms: Develop healthy coping mechanisms to deal with emotional triggers. Exercise, relaxation techniques like deep breathing or meditation, or spending time with loved ones can be helpful alternatives.

 * Don't Deprive Yourself: Complete deprivation can lead to intense cravings and binge eating. Allow yourself occasional treats in moderation to avoid feeling restricted.

 * Plan Ahead for Cravings: When cravings strike, have healthy alternatives readily available. Stock your pantry

with fruits, nuts, or Greek yogurt to satisfy cravings without derailing your goals.

 * Mindful Snacking: If you do choose to snack, practice mindful eating. Savor each bite and avoid mindless munching while distracted.

By understanding the root of cravings and emotional eating, endomorphs can develop strategies to manage these challenges and make healthier choices that support their weight management journey. In the next section, we'll discuss how to track progress and adjust your plan for optimal results.

Importance of tracking progress and adjusting the plan for endomorphs.

Here are some key points to consider:

* Monitoring Weight and Measurements: Regularly monitoring weight and body measurements can help you assess progress and identify plateaus. However, focus on overall health and body composition rather than just the scale.

* Track Food Intake: Keeping a food diary or using a calorie-tracking app can help you stay mindful of your portion sizes and identify areas for improvement in your diet.

* Non-Scale Victories: Celebrate non-scale victories like increased energy levels, improved mood, better sleep, or stronger muscles. These can be motivating indicators of progress.

* Adjusting Your Plan: As you progress, you may need to adjust your meal plan or exercise routine. A slight calorie decrease or tweaking your workout intensity might be necessary.

* Seek Support: Don't hesitate to seek support from a registered dietitian, certified personal trainer, or weight loss coach for guidance and motivation.

By tracking progress and being willing to adapt your plan, endomorphs can ensure their weight management approach remains effective and sustainable in the long term.

The following section can address frequently asked questions (FAQs) to provide further clarification and address common concerns endomorphs might have.

frequently asked questions

(FAQs) is a great way to provide further guidance and reassurance to endomorphs in the final section of your book. Here are some common questions you might encounter:

Q: Is it impossible for endomorphs to lose weight?

A: Absolutely not! While endomorphs may have a slower metabolism, weight loss is entirely achievable through a combination of a balanced diet, regular exercise, and mindful eating habits.

Q: Do endomorphs need to follow a strict, restrictive diet?

A: Restrictive diets are generally unsustainable and can be unhealthy. Endomorphs can achieve success with a balanced diet focused on whole foods, portion control, and adequate protein intake.

Q: What if I don't enjoy weight training?

A: Strength training is beneficial, but not the only option. Focus on finding physical activities you enjoy, whether it's dancing, swimming, or brisk walking. Consistency is key.

Q: How quickly can I expect to see results?
A: Weight loss is a gradual process. Focus on making sustainable changes and celebrate non-scale victories like increased energy or improved sleep.
Q: I keep getting cravings. What can I do?
A: Cravings are normal. Develop healthy coping mechanisms like exercise, relaxation techniques, or having healthy snacks on hand to avoid reaching for sugary or processed foods.
Q: What if I have a setback?
A: Everyone experiences setbacks. Don't get discouraged! Get back on track with your next meal and remember that progress, not perfection, is the goal.
By addressing these FAQs, you can empower endomorphs with the knowledge and confidence to achieve their weight management goals and embrace a healthy lifestyle.

Conclusion

Congratulations on completing this guide! You've taken a significant step towards a healthier and happier you. Remember, the key to success as an endomorph is to embrace a sustainable lifestyle that prioritizes your well-being. By incorporating the strategies outlined in this book, you can:
    * Manage your weight and improve body composition
 * Boost your metabolism and increase energy levels
 * Develop a healthy relationship with food
   * Cultivate a love for movement and physical activity
This journey is not about quick fixes or fad diets. It's about making gradual, positive changes that you can maintain for the long term. Trust the process, celebrate your victories, and don't be afraid to seek support and guidance when needed.
Here are some additional resources that you might find helpful:
 * Academy of Nutrition and Dietetics: Academy of Nutrition and Dietetics: https://www.eatright.org/
 * American Council on Exercise: American Council on Exercise: https://www.acefitness.org/
 * The National Institutes of Health (NIH): National Institutes of Health (NIH) Weight-Control Information Network: [invalid URL removed]

Remember, you are capable of achieving amazing things. Believe in yourself, and empower yourself to live a healthy and fulfilling life!

9 798325 693144